How to Lose Weight and Still Eat Everything you Want

Working with your food cravings

Julia Knight

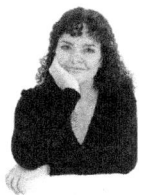

This book is dedicated to my amazing family, who have loved and supported me unconditionally, through thick and thin...

CONTENTS

INTRODUCTION

Congratulations, and thank you for purchasing this book.

So here we are again. You want to lose weight. You desperately want to lose weight, but you just can't stick to anything. Is there hope? Absolutely there is!

The first thing I look for when buying a book, is not qualifications, previous titles, celebrity endorsements or Facebook followers. All I really want to see is what the author looks like! Have they actually done it or are they just talking a good diet? Have they lost weight? Did they have a serious amount of weight to lose, or just felt overweight carrying an extra 5lbs? And where are their before and after pictures?

Whilst I do indeed have relevant qualifications, and I'm not a first-time author, as for the celebrity endorsement... I once helped push the broken-down car of the singer from The Commitments and there's a chance that he would've wished me well in this endeavour...

As for the before and after pictures, there are several in a later chapter.

There have been several changes since I decided to write this book. It started off as a general 'diet' book, to guide the reader through several workable regimes and to find one that suited. But the more I spoke to people, the more I realised that when we're struggling with our weight, what we really want to know is how to get into the right frame of mind. Most diets work, if we could only stick to them for longer than half an hour.

How do you diet when you just love eating so much? When you think about food as soon as you wake up? When the most important part of any planned excursion or activity is where and when you are going to eat?

It's all very well people saying "Just eat when you're hungry, and stop when you're full" I mean, why didn't I think of that? But what if you never get hungry because you've probably just eaten? And even if you're full, you can always find room for ice cream?

I've lost 10 stone - and I'd like to share with you how I did it.

Let me be clear, this is not a quick fix. You'll regularly take steps back as well as forwards, but you'll cross the finish line eventually. Then it won't feel like it took long at all .

I have tried to keep the science/biology 'aren't I clever?' bits to a minimum. Because if you've tried as many diets as I have, you already know all the theories, you just want it to work – regardless of why.

That's not to say that I don't know what I'm talking about. Not only am I now a fully qualified personal trainer, who has studied in nutrition along with many other qualifications. But, possibly more importantly, I have been where you are. Searching for something that works. For a book that understands me and doesn't just tell me what 'should' work, without the author having taken a single step in my shoes.

WHO IS THIS BOOK FOR?

This book was for me. This is the one I wish had been around for me to read when I was starting one of my many diet journeys, and when I realised that the way I approach diet and food didn't seem to fit with the advice I was being given.

I'm never going to be the sort of person who goes into a restaurant and gleefully orders a green salad and a sparkling water. That is not going out for dinner. You can have something miserable and boring at home. I wonder if it's just for show and they get home and order a family size pizza and a tub of Haagen Dazs?

And those pictures in magazines and on websites that show an apparent healthy option next to a chocolatey confection... they put a bright colourful fresh salad piled high on one side, then a Mars bar that's clearly had no sleep and has not been photographed from its best side, on the other. Me, I'm still having the Mars bar thanks.

If you are the type of person who orders the green salad and sparkling water – and actually WANTS to have that…. Step away from this book, this is not for you. You are just odd…

I realised that I can't be the only one who views food this way.

So, actually, this book is for us…

MINDSET - FIRST STEPS

- Make the decision
- Consult your doctor
- Set a goal
- Assemble your tools
- Choose a workable, sustainable, and enjoyable plan that you think you can follow

Make the decision

Start building up your enthusiasm. It won't be difficult – you do WANT to lose weight, don't you? Not just for your health, confidence, and appearance. But to feel able to live your life without being restricted or worried. And so that you can wear that size 12 sparkly dress that you bought 10 years ago. It may not be suitable for the supermarket, but, if it fits, we're wearing it, right?

If you have a serious weight problem, it is likely always going to be there. And when you've lost weight, you may always feel that you're on the verge of gaining it all back. However why not give it a whirl anyway? Lose the weight, feel amazing, be stronger and fitter than you ever have been and then you can work on staying there.

This will also be hard work, but you can do it, and more importantly, it will be worth it – very worth it. And wouldn't you rather be on the other side trying to stay there, than on this side, trying to get there?

Consult your doctor

Before starting any new regime, I advise talking to your doctor.

This is especially important if you have any other medical conditions that may be affected by a change in your diet. They may also give you some additional useful information for your goals such as blood pressure reading, cholesterol etc.

Set a goal

Setting a goal can be a bit tricky. You may think that a certain weight or size is what you're aiming for, but as you approach it, that may change.

That's okay. But you do need a goal first, then you can refine it as your new shape emerges. Make your goal somewhere in the healthy range for your age and height (oodles of info out there on this - but go by NHS apps or, even better, advice from your doctor).

To help you track your progress, weigh yourself at the same time, first thing in the morning, in the same (if any) clothes, on the same set of scales, in the same place every week. The accuracy of the scales isn't as important as you might think. It's the loss you are measuring, not the actual weight.

This is also worth bearing in mind if you go for any medical appointments where you are weighed. Their scales will show a different weight - do not let that distract you, regardless of whether they show an increase or decrease. I usually ask them not to tell me, and also avert my eyes.

Also take some measurements. You don't need to go to town on this. Just get a starting point on the main areas. Waist (and stomach, if, like me, your stomach is a separate entity in its own right). Chest, hips and upper arms and thighs. Preferably taken naked. Don't expect measurements to change as often as your weight, so don't measure every week. Leave it at least a month, or more.

And of course, you're going to need at least one 'before' photo. A word of warning on the photo - don't do it in the nude as you'll never be able to show anyone, and it will be the one photo that always pops up when you're flicking through your photos looking for that pair of shoes to show your friend...

Assemble your tools

So, you know where you are, and where you're heading. Now we need some tools to overcome all those pesky obstacles that are going to try to pull you off course.

'Stop Getting In Your Own Way' Also known as 'excuses'. Let's get them all out there and dealt with.

The only genuine acceptable excuse is "I don't really want to do it". Fine. I won't argue with that. Put this book down and carry on as you are...

For everything else - I'm going to be really irritating and come up with a counter-argument. These are your tools for coping with normal life, that won't stop just because you're on a diet.

I can't waste food: What do you consider to be a waste? Throwing food away? Okay, so will eating it be less of a waste? Will increasing the size of your stomach and the weight on the scales have made it less of a waste? Have you put it to better use by increasing your size? Can it be saved/chilled/frozen? If not, you have the choice of being fatter or throwing it away...?

I can't make different meals for everyone: Do you mean that you don't want to make different meals for everyone? That's fine - but you're getting in your own way! Find a solution that works for you. Prepare something that everyone will enjoy. Or pre-prepare either yours or theirs. Ask others to cook their own in order to help you (if old enough obviously). There are many ways around this, along with just putting yourself out for your own benefit and making different meals for everyone if that's the only thing that works.

We went out for dinner: It was still food and you still had a choice. The choice was probably more difficult and limited, and this can be a tough one to negotiate. But if you're determined, it can be overcome. For instance, you can always ask if you can have more vegetables instead of potatoes, or potatoes instead of chips. You don't have to have a bread roll if it's offered (no, it's not a waste). Even if it's a different cuisine, the same rules apply - ask for an alternative that's more in keeping with your regime. Or you could just have a smaller portion, or eat less of it. Of course, if it's a planned meal out - you can work it into a free day (more on this later).

You can also help yourself a lot by forward planning. For instance, if you're meeting a friend for a coffee and your chosen plan dictates a specific milk or cream - take some with you! You cannot expect that establishments will be able to cater for you and so you must think in advance. The world will not organise itself around your diet.

Gifts: This is a relatively easy one. Let's say it's a box of chocolates. You have two options. You can put them away for a free day (again, more on this later), or you can re-gift them. And if the gifter knew you were trying to lose weight - get a new friend.

At work: Another easy one. It can be really helpful to let the people that you work with know what you are trying to do. It will keep you accountable and people can be helpful. My own colleagues even managed not to glaze over in the face of many episodes of tedious diet talk. Take your own lunch in and make a massive diversion around any free roaming biscuits, chocolates, cakes etc, or put some in a sealable bag for a free day.

Evenings in front of the TV: This can be a tough one. The only way around this is to make sure that you have something else 'allowed' in your day to munch on later. Your chosen plan will dictate what this might be.

Personally, on a low carb plan I like to have corned beef slices, or crispy bacon strips, or Baby Bel cheeses. Failing that, another coffee with cream. You have to get to grips with this because evenings are not going anywhere, and neither is the TV (not in my house anyway).

Working away from home: This is easier than you might think. I have worked away many times and if I had used that as an excuse, I never would have reached my goal. It just takes thought and, yet again, planning.

On a recent work trip to Scotland, I was accompanied by a good friend and colleague, and we were staying in a hotel for two weeks. I was going to have to wing it. A challenge? Yes - but fortunately my friend was not only aware of my endeavours, but said she would have whatever I had.

So, we had a carb friendly breakfast every morning (so no beans or toast), went to the local supermarket for snacks (boiled eggs/bacon strips/sliced chicken) for lunch. Then we alternated between a 'picnic' of similar snacks in our hotel room, and a meal out in a restaurant, making careful choices like fish and extra vegetables, or a succulent lamb steak with mint sauce.

We certainly never went hungry, and we both lost weight!

Genetics: This one has been done to death. You may well be genuinely predisposed to weight gain, and may also find it far more difficult to lose weight than some other people. And you may also feel more hungry than other people. But, it can still be done, it just takes determination and the will to do it. It is going to be tough and I'm not making light of that. But no one can make these hurdles disappear. You can get over them, you just need to jump a little higher.

Birthday/Christmas/any other occasion: To be blunt, your body doesn't care what day of the year it is. If you eat too much you will gain weight regardless of the calendar. However, you can work around most of these occasions with your free days. Good planning is key. You will need a diary. Believe me when I say that if you manage to stick to your plan on one of these occasions, it will feel like a real achievement, and rightly so.

I work shifts: Working shifts can really mess with your body clock, and your determination can easily wane. So, it is really important to try to recognise when this is happening so that you can rescue yourself before you lose it. Have a few plans to fall back on. Something in the freezer that can be zapped quickly, a suitable snack that is always ready to go. If you eat a bit more to avoid a full-on slide, so be it. But not too regularly. And each time you overcome it, you will feel stronger next time.

But I'm on holiday: And I fully understand, that to really enjoy a holiday, it has to involve delicious food! But there are lots of delicious foods that you can have that aren't going to blow your entire plan.

It really is an incredible feeling to return from a holiday at either the same, or a lower weight! Remember - your body isn't going to ignore what you're eating just because you're away. And wouldn't it be great to be on holiday next year much lighter than you are now? Being able to open the plane table fully without it resting on your stomach? Lying on a sunbed without first inspecting it to see if it will hold your weight? A word of caution on alcohol - It is one of the quickest ways to lose all your good intentions - be warned!

You will of course have your own book of carefully crafted excuses. But all of them can be overcome by your desire to lose weight. Your attitude, common sense, and careful planning will get you through. You can do it!

Choose a workable, sustainable, and enjoyable plan that you think you can follow long term

Think about the types of food that you really enjoy eating. Write a list and then you should be able to see which diet will work best for you. Unfortunately, you are not going to find one that includes all the foods you love, all the time. It's a compromise between what you want, and what you're prepared to eat in order to get a designer body (designed by you).

WHICH DIETS WORK?

Almost every diet works! If you can stick to it. And there's the problem.

Doing the diet that the window cleaner's cousin did may well work for you, for a limited amount of time. But if you don't enjoy the foods you are eating, and just see it as a means to an end, then it will feel like a nightmarish slog and a constant battle.

Don't get me wrong, if it was as easy as pie (ooh pie...) then no-one would be overweight. But it can be less tough, and it absolutely must be sustainable for as long as it takes.

The one that works for you will be the one that you can stick to without feeling too restricted. It will likely involve a wide variety of foods to keep you interested for the long haul.

Yes of course it would be good if it also became a lifestyle but let's face it, if you overeat, that's unlikely to completely disappear. The type of diet that you want to do has to suit you and your tastes.

As it's my personal advice being offered here, I'm going to talk mainly about a low carbohydrate diet but if you are going to be miserable without bread rice potatoes et cetera, then you need to follow a different regime to create meals that you will enjoy using the ingredients that fit with your diet choice. So, if, for example, you decide to go low-fat you need to write a list of delicious allowable options to get you fired up and off the starting blocks.

Although there are probably, what seems like, about 5.7 billion diets out there. They mostly fall into three broad categories: Calorie Controlled, Low Fat and Low Carbohydrate.

Calorie controlled dieting: Count everything! Calorie counting is a good way to get used to the amounts and types of food that you can eat. You won't always have to count everything, but to start with, it will be your guide.

When you are very overweight, you don't tend to get, or respond in the normal way to hunger signals. You've either never stopped eating long enough to get hungry, or been on such a severe diet that you learn to ignore them. So relying on your hunger signals when you start on a different eating regime may not work – this is where calories can help.

Consume less calories than you use. So, add up all your calories for a normal '**non-diet**' day. Everything includes little extras like biscuits or mints served with coffee, the bits you eat from the kid's plates as you clear the dishes, all drinks except plain water, – EVERY SINGLE THING! Write it down in a book or on a piece of paper, and record it at the time. Don't try to remember it later – that never works.

You may need to do this over several days, or a week if your intake fluctuates a lot. No judgments here - no-one is seeing this except you. But you need a realistic start point, so don't miss writing anything down.

Now you need to work out a sensible daily allowance. Whatever your 'normal' calorie intake is, reduce that by 500 per day. When you're used to consuming a lot of calories, you may have to experiment to find the point at which your body lets go of body weight. So, if you don't lose weight at this, then reduce again until you find the amount that leads to a 1lb or 2lbs loss per week.

There are many BMR (Basal Metabolic Rate) apps and tools and calculators out there that claim to tell you how many calories your body is burning a day. And these can give you some guidance, but the most personalised way to do it, is by trialling it yourself. This gives you a custom framework to start from.

You may also have to adjust this amount every so often as you get lighter. I quite like calorie-controlled diets as they are very flexible. You can eat whatever you want to - but only up to your calorie limit. Calorie information is available on just about everything you consume, and in some restaurants too.

You could, in theory, eat several Mars bars per day (other yummy chocolate confections are available) up to your limit. But actually, this doesn't really work out so well (yes of course I've tried it!). Because you eat all the chocolate far too early in the day leaving nothing for later when you crash back down from the sugar rush. Not forgetting the obvious - this is not a particularly healthy way to eat!

So, you will probably start to seek out foods that fill you up for less calories. This can be a good thing, as it often leads to vegetables, fish, chicken etc. And there are some really tasty ready meals available too and all calorie counted.

Never drop your calories to less than an absolute minimum of 1,250 per day. If your normal intake is already less than 1,750 and so cannot be dropped by 500, then you can drop the calories to 1,250, but will need to accept a slower loss.

However, more importantly, you may need to consult a doctor if you are obese and not losing weight on 1,250 calories.

Low fat: Low fat diets used to be the 'go to' diet for most people. Fat was seen as the bad guy, and to be fair it does have more calories than either protein or carbohydrates (Fat = 9 cals per gram, both protein and carbs have 4, and alcohol has 7). But we do need an amount of healthy fats in our diet to enable us to absorb certain vitamins, support cell growth, protect our organs and keep us warm.

As with the calorie-controlled diet, you need to find the 'sweet spot' at which your body reacts to fat reduction. It is counted in grammes per day. So again, write down everything on a normal non-diet day in order to find a start point for your changes. Then reduce the fat grams you eat until you start to lose weight at 1-2lbs per week.

As you can see, there are some similarities in these two regimes, and when you cut through all the hype and over-complications, the basic premise is easy to implement.

Low Carbohydrate: This is the diet that suited me, and that I not only managed to stick to throughout my weight loss campaign, but that I still stick to because I can!

Again, we are reducing a food group. This time, obviously, carbohydrates. There are quite a few variations to be found, but basically, there is low carb, and then there is very low carb which is often called 'Keto' short for 'Ketogenic'. Don't get too concerned about the names. We are going to start with low carb, with the option, further down the line of fine-tuning with keto.

As with low fat and calorie-controlled regimes, we are first seeking that point at which your body will start to lose weight. So, no surprises here, you need to do the same sort of food diary to establish 'your normal intake'.

I'm going to give you a bit of a goal here. Try to get down to 100g of carbs per day. This may be tougher than you think. But remember, at this point, we are not counting calories.

Next aim for 75g, and then maybe 50g, depending on how you are doing. If you are losing weight steadily at 100g, then stick with that as it gives you somewhere to go when you plateau.

I don't want you to worry too much about calories at this stage. And don't be afraid of fat! It makes things taste nice and so you feel more satisfied after eating.

Good fats like Olive oil, Avocados, Salmon, Nuts (but watch the carbs) are healthy and contribute to HDL (good cholesterol). But avoid artificial trans-fats like the plague! Check food labels and avoid anything with trans-fats or hydrogenated vegetable oil.

If, as you lose weight you get to a point where you're not losing for a few weeks, and you have reduced your carbs to 50g, then you could consider going full keto and reducing your carbs to 20g per day, with fat making up around 70-80% of your daily intake.

By the time you get to looking at this you'll hopefully be well on your way anyway, and as I keep saying - this is fine-tuning for further down the line.

Now unfortunately I'm not saying that you can eat as much as you want on low carb, and some people can over-do it. But you only really need to start to look at calorie intake if you aren't progressing.

There are many, many books and articles written on low carb, and it is fast becoming recognised as a healthy way to eat, and even to reduce insulin resistance which causes a lot of over-weight people to genuinely struggle more than most to both lose weight and keep it off. I said "struggle" though - not "find it impossible" So no using that as an excuse!

Diets in Summary; You don't need me to tell you how many diets there are out there. You've probably tried a fair few of them, lost weight, and then found it all again with interest.

But regardless of all the different names, they still mainly fall into the categories I've mentioned. There are also different timings, and fasting regimes etc. These are all things that you can experiment with when the bulk of the work is done if you want to.

Whichever you choose, try to make sure you have a good variety of different foods so that you will get plenty of different nutrients and vitamins and won't get easily bored. It will then be more sustainable and enjoyable.

Make wise choices when faced with a decision. Choose the best of two evils if you have to. Every little good decision you make, will pay you back.

I'd like to add a word for people with specific dietary requirements. Whether these are due to personal choices, ethical concerns, animal welfare, religious reasons, or food allergies.

The person who is the best expert on these matters - is you. You have either had to live with, or chosen to live with, these requirements. And although I have trained in nutrition and could tell you how to get all your different protein requirements, for me to tell you what you can and cannot eat would be frankly, a bit patronising.

I usually find that people with such specific requirements are amongst the most organised when it comes to their eating. Often armed with alternatives, and scrupulous at checking ingredients.

So, my advice is the same. Pick whichever diet you feel you can work with the best. I would think that if you are vegan, you may find low carb the most difficult. That's not to say that you can't do it - but your options may be more limited.

Low fat should not cause too many problems, and calorie controlled is of course the most flexible. There are some great plant-based products and ready meals available too. As I'm sure you already know.

I could have written pages and pages on which diets are out there, but you don't need that. That's been done time and time again, and there is no requirement for me sticking my oar in too. Which is why I've tried to keep it concise and relevant to the real issue we have - sticking to it - whatever 'it' you choose.

For now - pick one and stick with it. You can't for example do low carb for three days and low-fat for four. There is no mix and match. Pick one!

It's possible that in the first few weeks you may lose more as you release water stored with energy sources. This is completely normal (and a nice boost). But overall, be patient.

It took me 100 weeks to lose 123lbs. I then reassessed my goals, and lost a further 17lbs - at my leisure. I am now comfortable at my current healthy weight. And if I start drifting, I reign it in before it gets out of hand.

WHAT DID I DO DIFFERENTLY THIS TIME?

When I have lost weight previously (low fat diet) and got close to a goal, it had been so difficult that I couldn't wait to be off it. I maintained that 'close to goal' weight for about 10 minutes.

This time, I took into account the reasons why I fail. It's because I binge eat. I eat when I'm not hungry, I eat when I'm full, I eat chocolate/cake/crisps etc at any time of the day. I don't reserve cereals for breakfast, and treats for the evening. I won't just have one bowl of cereal/1 bar of chocolate/a couple of biscuits - I'll keep going back for more, and more. But if it tasted so good the first time, why wouldn't you want to eat it again? Does this sound familiar?

But what about just "eat less, move more"? That is good and sensible advise, and is in the end what you have to do. But your mindset must be changed first, otherwise it's just more twee sound-bites that don't really help, and are usually dished out by someone who hasn't had a serious weight problem.

But let's face the truth - you are going to have to eat less. But for me, facing a future with no glorious feasts, and no lattes and no cakes was just never going to work.

I couldn't, and evidently didn't, commit to that, time and time again. A hard slog stretching out in front of me with no reprieve for good behaviour? I tried, and tried, and tried. I just couldn't do it. So, sad though it may sound...I needed the binges.

You have to recognise your faults and weaknesses and then work out how to adjust your behaviours and work with them. Here's exactly what I did...

Of the vast array of diets to choose from, I decided that I could build up the most enthusiasm for a low carb diet. Less counting, especially in the early phases. Lots of foods that I absolutely love and could look forward to. Plenty of options for eating out, and lots of foods that aren't found on other restrictive regimes.

For example:

Salmon and broccoli drizzled with butter
Bacon, fried eggs, sausages and mushrooms
Chicken legs with crispy skin
Ribeye steak with mushrooms, tomato and butter
Sliced ham with cheese and mayonnaise
Sugar-free jelly with double cream
Duck legs with veg and butter
Egg mayonnaise salad
Prawn and avocado salad
Just prawns and rose-marie sauce
Coffee with cream

Call that a diet? Actually, I do.

So far, so good. But I need/want other, less wholesome things. So, here's the deal; Every half stone that I lose (7lbs) I will have a day off. Completely off. No limits, no counting, no mental notes, no recording, and most importantly - no guilt!

I will weigh every Friday, and after reaching at least a 7lbs loss, I will plan my day off, usually a Saturday. I say usually because I would sometimes use this day for a special occasion like a party, birthday, meal out, a trip to the cinema that just HAS to include chocolate/popcorn etc.

This is where your planning comes in again - if something is approaching, take control and include it. Plan for days off. This way, nothing is ever banned - it's just delayed or put on hold until it fits.

Now you may well ask, and you certainly should be asking, but doesn't this day off lead to a weight gain? Yes it does. And it would usually take me three weeks to get back to where I was, along with an additional slight loss. But - I was still following the regime, I was still on course, I hadn't 'broken my diet'.

Instead of seeing an endless stretch of fighting to resist everything I love in front of me, I was just setting off on course for the next free day.

Therefore, you should only aim to be losing an average of around 1lb a week. Some weeks will be a gain, some may be a good loss. But on average, set yourself up for expecting 1lb per week. Anything more is a bonus.

Remember that I lost 123lbs in 100 weeks. It may sound like a small amount per week, but it certainly adds up. Think of it as two steps forward, one step back.

This may sound counter-intuitive, and obviously you would lose weight quicker not having the free days - but would you stick to it? If not, then you're not losing any weight!

I never call this day off a 'cheat day' because I'm not cheating. It's built into my plan. It's either a day off or a free day. It's much easier sticking to a plan for an extended amount of time if you can actually persevere. That's why when I'd reached my original 'goal' I was able to stick with it to get down further, rather than being desperate to ditch the diet.

Having the attitude that nothing was banned helped me in so many ways. If I had a craving for something, I would add it to my shopping or write it down. Yes, I can have it on my next free day.

Cravings will not go away for long whether you give in to them or not. So you may as well resist until it's controlled and on your terms. That cake possibly will taste as good as you imagine... But you'll still want it again the following week/day/hour. I would say that it's not going anywhere, but I once thought that about a vanilla and raspberry cake in Costa, and by the time I allowed myself to have it, it was no longer available as it was a limited edition! I still want that cake...

Now the day after a free day can be either a relief or really difficult. But remember, another one will be along soon, and you'll be another half stone lighter by then.

Is this healthy? I think it's reasonably obvious that a healthier plan would not include the free days. But we have to balance best practice with a healthy outcome.

Is it healthy to be as overweight as you currently are? And your risks are increasing the longer you stay at that weight. My method may be a little unusual/controversial, but if you end up lighter and healthier by doing it, then the end result will be worth it.

Our bodies were created to be able to function during feast or fast. And while it may feel strange - it's not that far removed. Although I'm not sure that Neanderthal Man had access to McDonalds, Thorntons or Deliveroo (other takeaways, confectioners, and delivery services are doubtless available).

As I have already said elsewhere. Please talk to your doctor before embarking on a new diet or exercise plan. This is especially important if you have any other health issues.

Please also consider that the very fact that you are here reading this book could be pointing to a serious issue with food and the possibility of an eating disorder. If you think this is affecting you, help is available out there - please talk to someone.

BUT YOU HAVEN'T MENTIONED EXERCISE

Well, been as you've brought it up! Exercise is fabulous. In almost every way and in almost every case, exercise is beneficial. Even a tiny bit of additional movement (dancing to a favourite song, going upstairs even when there's no cake up there) will give you health gains, both visible and invisible.

Exercise will improve your cardiovascular system, your muscles, your state of mind, your balance, strength, and endurance. It will make your body more efficient at using the fuel you give it and give shape to your body.

All good right? YES! All good. But are you going to start your new regime if I tell you that you must do it?

Your diet will make the most difference to your weight. You can't out-train a bad diet. Going for a walk is not going to make up for something you didn't plan to eat. It will do lots of other good stuff - but it won't work 'instead'.

Of course, if you want to include an existing or new fitness regime, absolutely do it. You may also find that as you start to lose weight and feel better, you will actually want to get more active. This is the best time to start, when your enthusiasm and energy is pushing you to do it, rather than me trying to drag you kicking and screaming into a leotard.

I have added an additional chapter at the end of this book focusing on getting started when you're totally unfit. When you feel ready... take a look.

WHEN SHOULD I START?

It's all very well me saying "start now" but your start date needs to suit you. You need to get yourself fired up and enthusiastic. You need to *want* to get going. Only you know when you've had enough of lugging around your current weight. That's when you should take control.

'Diet' has negative connotations which are not deserved. Some dictionary definitions of 'diet' are: "The kinds of food that a person, animal or community habitually eats" and "Food and drink considered in terms of its qualities, composition, and its effects on health" I can't find a definition that says "Makes you miserable."

Your mindset is the main thing that will determine your success and push you to make the decision. Live with that decision, plant it and let it grow in your mind. Start to imagine being on your new journey and coping with it. Build on it every day. Start writing your food diary.

Think about the food that you are really going to enjoy and look forward to eating on your diet. Write a list of delicious foods like the one I did for low carb. Choose foods that you would enjoy whether you were on a diet or not. It must be foods that you love not just foods that work for someone else. You can't make yourself suddenly like the meals on a diet if you wouldn't like them otherwise. This would not be sustainable and would lead to another very short-lived tortuous failed diet. So, get revved up, get excited about the food that you're going to be able to enjoy. Don't allow yourself to eat them before you start, make it like a treat, something to look forward to. Build the anticipation until you just can't wait to get started.

You will need to write stuff down! Get into a firm habit of writing stuff down. I did a simple table in Excel and printed out several blank tables at a time then filled them in manually (with an actual pen). This table changed over time as each stage of my weight loss needed changes and tweaks to my macros (protein/fat/carbs) which is why I only printed out a few at a time with maybe 4-7 days on each side of the pages. It doesn't have to be a table - you can just write it all down. Even when using a tracker app (more on that in a moment), still write it down. Just go with me on this - it works.

I have included a few examples of what I did, but you will find your own best way. I would also strongly recommend that you use a tracker app to track your food diary. There are quite a few to choose from including Fat Secret and MyFitnessPal. People tend to find their favourite one just by using them and seeing which features work for them. I personally use Nutracheck. Most are either completely free, or have a free trial, so you can see which one you 'gel' with. It has to be able to show your food intake summary in calories, fat, protein and carbs. Then you are set up for whichever diet you follow, and also for any tweaking later on as your shape changes.

Get your before photos and measurements done as well. You may wish to get a set of scales that also measures other things such as body fat (for guidance only), which are relatively inexpensive, but this is in no way essential - and don't switch scales after you've started! The wailing and moaning that will ensue just isn't worth it. Same scales for the duration! We're measuring the loss, not the exact, to the ounce, weight.

Now... are you ready? GO!

IDEAS FOR LOW CARB

Per day:
Coffee x 3 with cream – or tea, made with whole milk
Latte – Medium latte or home-made milky coffee with whole milk
Lunch – Two small items, examples below
Dinner – examples below
2 x snack items – Examples below
2 x 75 calories – Self-explanatory, but suggest use for vegetables with dinner
No meals or snacks after 8pm
Drinks can be drunk at any time
First drink/snack/meal of day at your own discretion
Try to avoid any additional carbs (don't use extra calories on bread or fruit)

Example lunch and snack items (all = 1 selection):
Kefir quark
2 slices corned beef (optional mayonnaise)
Boiled egg
4-5 rashers crispy dried bacon
Handful of unsalted cashews/walnuts/pecans etc
Coffee with tablespoon of double cream
100% chocolate (small amount – about 15g)
2 mini peperami sticks
Babybel cheese
Kefir quark

Dinner examples:

2 fried eggs, 3 rashers of bacon fried in coconut butter

Smoked haddock in cheese sauce

3 egg omelette

Lamb steak

Cheesy chicken – Large curl of butter in small baking tin, salt & pepper, chicken breast on top, more seasoning if wanted, cover with grated mature cheddar. Cook on 160 (fan) for 36 mins.

Steak and mushrooms

Chicken with or without skin

Vegetables drizzled with butter and/or cheese

AVOID – Bread, fruit, rice, pasta, potatoes. Anything high in carbs – there are enough in the milk, veg, nuts. Avoid any added sugar.

Be very careful with supposed 'healthy' labelled foods. For instance, a low fat yoghurt may contain much more sugar than a creamy greek style yoghurt, and therefore more carbs. The same applies to milk - full fat is better for low carb (or cream). So read the labels and get familiar with which specific information you need for your chosen diet.

These suggestions are for guidance only. Just to give you some ideas if you're struggling with where to start. You will find your own routines and favourites, regardless of which type of diet you decide to follow. Remember – most diets will work if you can stick to them.

NOTES, TABLES, AND PICTURES FROM MY OWN JOURNEY...

Over the next few pages, you will see a blank grid for five days with some suggestion headings for low carb. Also a few of my own filled-in grids. As you will see, I change things as I go. I was having red wine every day, but then changed that to a latte. I now only have coffee with cream in as it's much lower in carbs.

On the blank one I have also put boxes for additional entries like % of Fats/Carbs/Protein, and on all of them there is a box for exercise. The exercise box is more of a reminder for me to do some! Do not attempt to eat exercise calories. That two-minute walk around the living room does not equal a bag of crisps – or probably even a crisp.

Apologies for all the scribbles, but I didn't know at the time that I would be publishing them!

Please remember that this is guidance only, and clearly skewed towards low carb. But you can customise your own food choices to suit you. This is not intended to be a specific diet – more a diet style.

I have also included some before and after photographs of me, which I hope will inspire you.

I remember thinking so many times that I would never get there. I did, so can you...

Coffee with cream

Latte

Lunch

Dinner

2 x snack items

Misc

Exercise

Cals:
Carbs:

%

Fat:

Protein:

Carbs:

Coffee with cream

Latte

Lunch

Dinner

2 x snack items

Misc

Exercise

Cals:
Carbs:

%

Fat:

Protein:

Carbs:

Coffee with cream

Latte

Lunch

Dinner

2 x snack items

Misc

Exercise

Cals:
Carbs:

%

Fat:

Protein:

Carbs:

Coffee with cream

Latte

Lunch

Dinner

2 x snack items

Misc

Exercise

Cals:
Carbs:

%

Fat:

Protein:

Carbs:

Coffee with cream

Latte

Lunch

Dinner

2 x snack items

Misc

Exercise

Cals:
Carbs:

%

Fat:

Protein:

Carbs:

Daily

Coffee x 3 *Latte*

Latte

Lunch = 2 x snack items *Latte*

Dinner *Cheesy chicken*

2 x snack items *Nuts/chocolate*

2 x half glasses red wine *(Home Latte)*

Hot milk

Exercise calories

+1

Monday (travel srs)

Daily

Coffee x 3

Latte

Lunch = 2 x snack items

Dinner *Chicken leg.*

2 x snack items *Nuts/chocolate*

2 x half glasses red wine *(Home latte)*

Hot milk

Exercise calories

42+3 = 1 be

Tuesday

Daily

Coffee x 3

Latte *(Home)*

Lunch = 2 x snack items *Quark/nuts*

Dinner *Chicken leg*

2 x snack items *Nuts/chocolate*

2 x half glasses red wine *(Home latte)*

Hot milk

Yoghurt or kefir - optional

Exercise calories

Wednesday

Daily

Coffee x 3

Latte *(Home)*

Lunch = 2 x snack items *Quark*

Dinner *Smoked haddock*

2 x snack items *Nuts/chocolate*

2 x half glasses red wine *(Home latte)*

Hot milk

Yoghurt or kefir - optional

Exercise calories

Thursday
~~Friday~~

Daily
Coffee x 3
Latte
Lunch = 2 x snack items
Dinner *Bacon & eggs*
2 x snack items *Nuts / chocolate*
2 x half glasses red wine
Hot milk

Exercise calories *138*

Friday
~~Bacon~~

Daily
Coffee x 3 *Latte*
Latte
Lunch = 2 x snack items *Coffee (creamy) Nuts*
Dinner *Bacon & eggs*
2 x snack items *Babybel /*
2 x half glasses red wine
Hot milk

Exercise calories

Saturday
Daily
Coffee x 3 *Latte*
Latte *Latte*
Lunch = 2 x snack items *Latte (Home)*
Dinner *Omelette (3 eggs)*
2 x snack items *Nuts / chocolate*
2 x half glasses red wine *(ran out)*
Hot milk
~~Yoghurt or kefir - optional~~

Exercise calories *150*

Sunday
Daily
Coffee x 3 *Latte*
Latte ~~x2~~
Lunch = 2 x snack items *Latte*
Dinner *Haddock*
2 x snack items *Nuts / chocolate*
2 x half glasses red wine *Latte (home)*
Hot milk
~~Yoghurt or kefir - optional~~

Exercise calories *149*

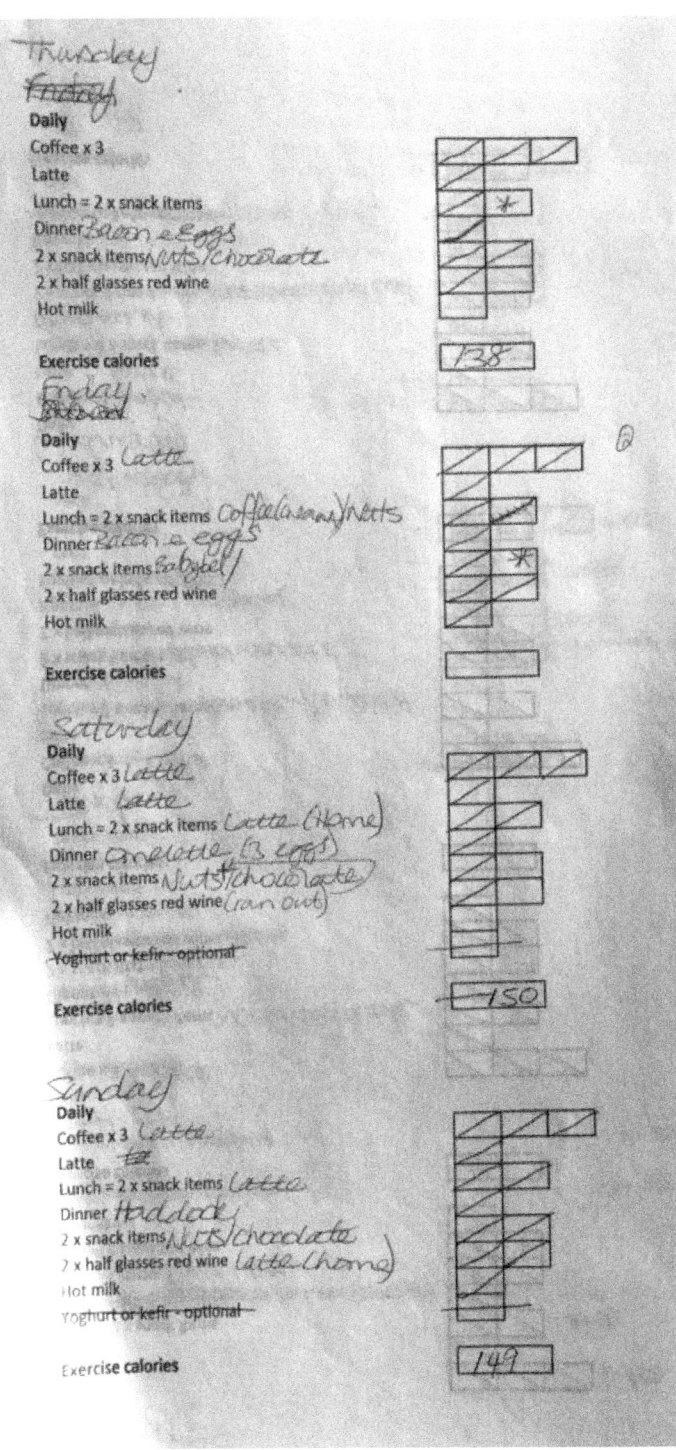

Tuesday 24th
Daily
Coffee x 3
Latte Home
Lunch = 2 x snack items Quark/Nuts
Dinner Bacon e Eggs
2 x snack items Chocolate
2 x half glasses red wine (Home latte)
Hot milk

Exercise calories 139

Wednesday 25th
Daily
Coffee x 3
Latte Costa
Lunch = 2 x snack items Quark/Nuts
Dinner Bacon e Eggs
2 x snack items Chocolate
2 x half glasses red wine (Home Latte)
Hot milk

Exercise calories

Thursday 26th
Daily
Coffee x 3
Latte Home
Lunch = 2 x snack items Quark/Nuts
Dinner Cheesy Chicken
2 x snack items Chocolate
2 x half glasses red wine (Home Latte)
Hot milk
Yoghurt or kefir - optional

Exercise calories 153

Friday
Daily
Coffee x 3
Latte Home
Lunch = 2 x snack items Latte (Costa) x3
Dinner Cheesy chicken
2 x snack items Chocolate/Nuts
2 x half glasses red wine (Home Latte)
Hot milk
Yoghurt or kefir - optional

Exercise calories 145

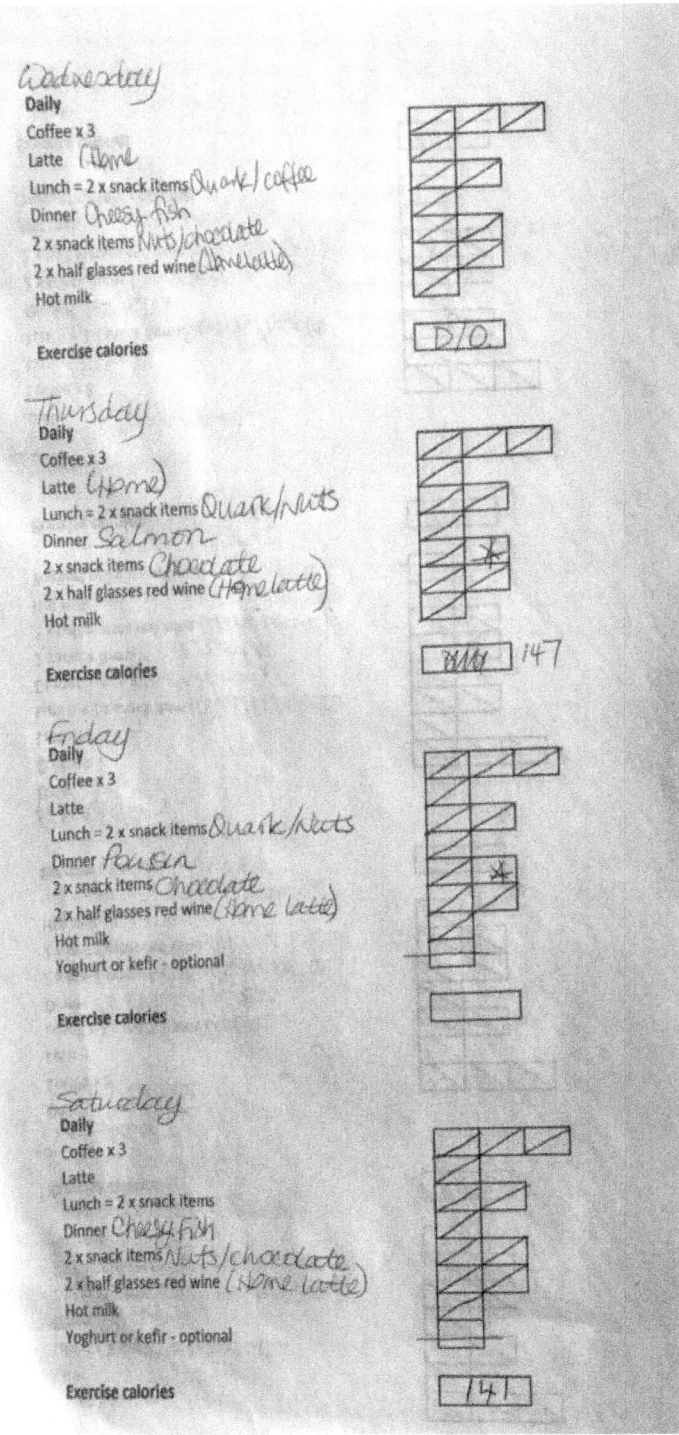

Wednesday

Daily

Coffee x 3

Latte (Home

Lunch = 2 x snack items Quark/coffee

Dinner Cheesy fish

2 x snack items Nuts/chocolate

2 x half glasses red wine (Home latte)

Hot milk

Exercise calories

D/O

Thursday

Daily

Coffee x 3

Latte (Home)

Lunch = 2 x snack items Quark/nuts

Dinner Salmon

2 x snack items Chocolate

2 x half glasses red wine (Home latte)

Hot milk

Exercise calories

147

Friday

Daily

Coffee x 3

Latte

Lunch = 2 x snack items Quark/nuts

Dinner Pousin

2 x snack items Chocolate

2 x half glasses red wine (Home latte)

Hot milk

Yoghurt or kefir - optional

Exercise calories

Saturday

Daily

Coffee x 3

Latte

Lunch = 2 x snack items

Dinner Cheesy fish

2 x snack items Nuts/chocolate

2 x half glasses red wine (Home latte)

Hot milk

Yoghurt or kefir - optional

Exercise calories

141

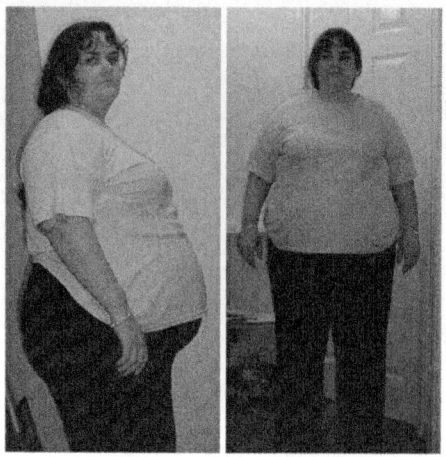

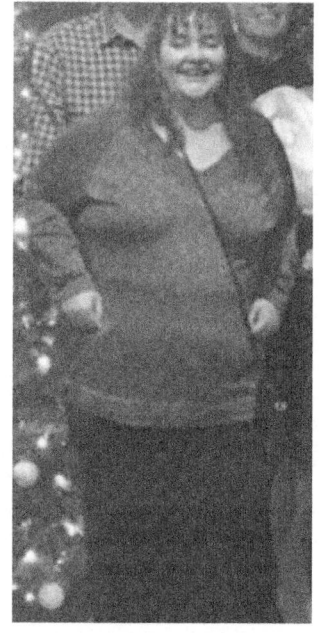

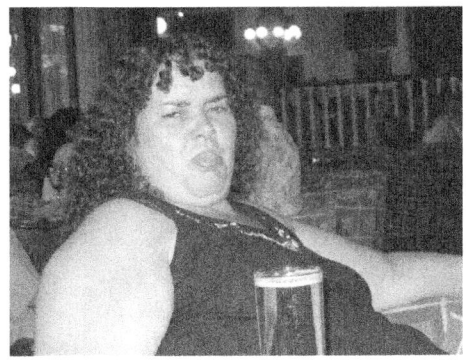

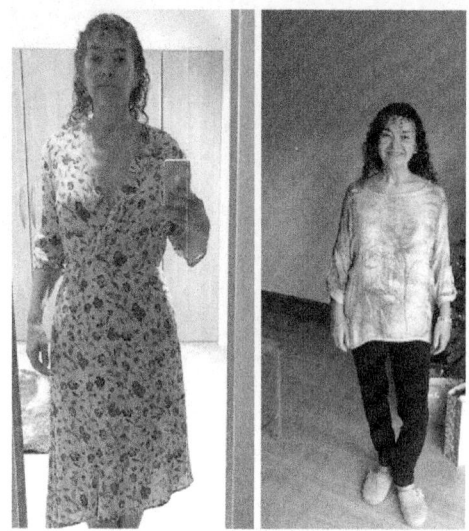

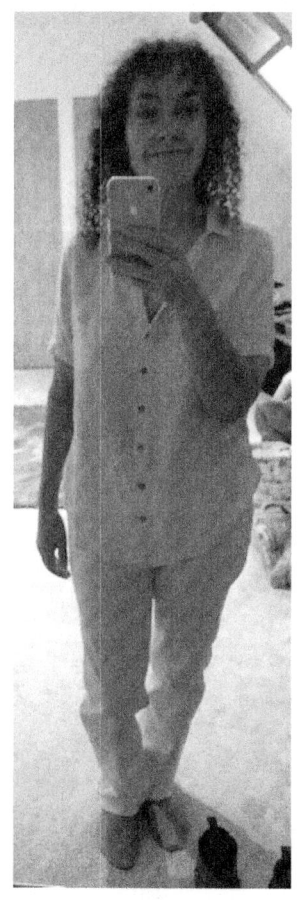

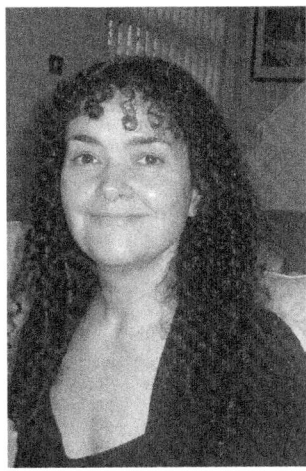

THE ROAD AHEAD

It is going to take a while. I can't change that. And despite the ever-present hype, no one else can either. But although the road may be long, the scenery changes as you go. Here are just a few things to look forward to along your journey:

Driving your car without your stomach rubbing against the steering wheel

Not worrying about restaurant seating being strong enough or big enough

Being able to sit in snuggly chairs, maybe with your legs curled under you, instead of being jammed in

Getting in and out of the shower opening just one door

Reaching the kitchen window as your stomach is no longer fighting with the sink

The blood pressure cuff at doctors is the 'normal' sized one instead of extra-large! And as you would expect, a lower blood pressure too

Wearing thick jumpers under your coat, and layers without looking like the Michelin Man

Actively looking at your refection in shop windows without grimacing

Buying new clothes - but don't buy clothes in a smaller size – they never look right as your shape changes. Buy clothes for the shape you are when you buy them

Realising that you are no longer the fattest person in the pool/shop/café/Universe

I recently bought a bicycle, and as I was searching the information for the maximum weight it would carry, it ocurred to me that I was very unlikely to exceed it! But out of habit, it was one of the first things I looked for.

These are the kinds of things that someone who has never had a weight problem would not even think about, but I add things all the time, and they regularly make me smile.

What would also make me smile, is if this book helps others to be free of the weight, and feel as wonderful as I do now.

WHERE TO START WHEN YOU'RE TOTALLY UNFIT...

This chapter is aimed at people who are trying to get to that first basic level of fitness and need guidance on how to get there.

I've put this guide together based on the most common questions that I get asked, and I'll start with:

Am I too heavy to start exercising?

A lot of people think that they need to lose some weight before they can begin to exercise, this is not the case, and the sooner you start, the sooner you will see and feel the benefits.

Do I need to join a gym?

No. Of course, you can if you want to, but it certainly isn't essential. There are some exercise choices that may mean you need a gym, leisure centre or specific venue such as swimming, squash, or kayaking, but there are plenty of things you can do. The choice is yours, if you do something that you enjoy, you are more likely to keep doing it. It's a good idea to try a few different forms of exercise to see what you enjoy. You may like to be in a class situation, or you may prefer to go it alone. The good news is that there is plenty of variety.

Do I need equipment?

Yes, a pair of trainers! Unless of course your chosen exercise is swimming.

How soon will I feel the benefit?

The benefits of exercise happen very quickly. From the first session, there will be positive health effects happening in your body. As you continue, your heart and lungs will be getting stronger, more oxygen will be delivered to your working muscles and you will become more efficient at doing the exercise.

Am I too old to start exercising?

No! Age is no barrier to exercise and is beneficial to all age groups. As with everyone, you should always consult your doctor before you embark on an exercise plan, so that you know you are safe to proceed.

Will I be able to eat more?

Unfortunately not. You can't out-train a bad diet. It needs to be a side-by-side effort of both training and diet. You can consume far more calories with a little extra snack than you're likely to have used during exercise. But there are far more additional benefits that you gain from exercise than just using up calories.

Should I take medical advice before I start?

Yes, absolutely. You must consult your doctor to make sure that it's safe for you to start exercising. This will also reassure you.

So, once you've made the decision, and been cleared by your doctor, what do you do next?

Having a goal is especially important. It doesn't have to be a huge goal, just something to work towards. For instance, your first one could be to run for 10 mins, walk a mile, swim 10 lengths or cycle 3 miles.

I've based this on running (or shuffling, if my first steps are anything to go by), but it can be used for many other activities such as walking, swimming, or cycling. If you are very overweight, your doctor may advise starting with walking or swimming to lessen the stress on your joints. Or they may not! But follow advice.

Get into your trainers and comfortable clothes, appropriate to the weather. Make sure nothing's going to flap around you and be distracting. Spend a few minutes warming up - what I mean by this is doing actions that you are going to be doing during the exercise and preparing your body.

So, for our run, marching on the spot is a good warm up - also briefly stretch your arms forward and back several times and roll your shoulders, but there's no need to hold theses stretches, we just want to prepare the muscles and joints, not stretch them out completely.

Now, this first outing is to put a base line in place, a benchmark to measure future sessions against, so that you have something to work towards. The most basic way to record your performance will be either to time the run, or to make a mental note of where you got to. A watch with a timer on would be helpful, and personally I like to listen to music while running, so if you have an iPod or similar, you may find it helps. Of course, you can get all sorts of extras like apps for your phone and GPS tracking etc that will chart your running distance, time, and speed, but let's not get away from the very basics, let's just concentrate on getting out there first.

When I ventured out for my first stagger, I was intending to run around the block - I didn't know how far that was, but it seemed quite short in the car. I got as far as the second lamppost round the first corner. It was a grand total of 2 minutes 40 seconds! I was beetroot red, embarrassed in case the neighbours could see me, and determined never to try it again!

So, it really doesn't matter how far you get, because another great thing about exercise Is how quickly you can improve. And as soon as you go out on that second run, and get further than your last marker, you realise that it is possible, that you can improve and that it really doesn't matter where you start, it just matters that you start!

So walk out of your door, don't feel embarrassed - you're out there doing something, you should feel proud. Take small steps, rather than long strides, try not to cross your arms in front of your body, try to have good control over your body, hold your posture, don't slouch, try not to land too heavily, and aim to get into a rhythm. It may seem like a lot to try to remember, but while you're busy thinking about all that, your feet are moving and you're covering ground.

Listen to your body. This doesn't mean that as soon as it gets hard going and you're sweating a bit it's time to stop. It means that you should be aware of danger signals - difficulty breathing, chest pains, dizziness. Make no mistake, you should be working hard, and it won't be easy, but you must know the difference between hard work and danger signals.

When you've gone as far as you can, you can either take a breather by walking a little then running again or walk back home from where you are. If you are running, when you get back, walk around a little before stopping completely, as a sudden stop can lead to feelings of light headedness due to your blood pooling in your legs. This is normal and can be easily prevented by stopping gradually.

A good stretch out of the muscles you've been using would be beneficial, holding a stretch this time and really feeling them loosening off.

You now have a starting point, either a physical marker such as a lamppost or house number, or a time on your watch. If you're using the time method, remember that at this stage we're not looking to do the same distance in a shorter time, we're looking to increase the time that you're running.

When you get this far, you've taken that enormous first step.

And you've set the bar for next time. Well done! There's no reason why you should ever look back.

Ideally, to start, you should try to get out every other day if possible. If not, fit it in where you can, but try not to bunch it up by doing 3 or 4 days consecutively and nothing for the rest of the week. Keep it regular.

You don't have to get further or for longer than the last time each and every day you go out, you will have good and bad days, and these can be caused by so many things such as sleep patterns, diet, and general mood. But you're still strengthening your heart and lungs, still having positive effects on your body and still burning calories!

So now you're wondering if you're going to have to just keep going further or longer every time and end up running for hours on end?

Well, no, you're not, unless you decide that you want to train for a specific running event like a marathon. You're just building up your base fitness level.

When you can run for a couple of miles, or 20-30 minutes with relative ease then you can start looking at the next steps. You can start adding in intervals, steps, hills etc. You may decide to keep at that running level and add in another activity like Kettlebells or boxing!

Once you start to feel the strength from training you may find you become interested in all sorts of other exercises.

There are plenty of people in the gym that are on the treadmill for an hour or two, at the same pace, doing the same thing week in week out. You really don't need to get into that sort of tedious routine. Variety is far more effective for fitness and fat fighting, and fortunately, there's plenty of variety out there.

So there you have the very first steps

Medical clearance
Trainers
Leave your home or place of work
Put one foot in front of the other
Create a benchmark and have a goal
Get there

I've used running in this plan, but as you can see, you can apply the same principles to say, cycling, walking or swimming.

Taking that first step can be daunting, but you can take your trainers anywhere, and wherever your feet can come into contact with the ground, you can run or walk. And yes, that does include marching or running on the spot indoors, although being out-doors will be far more enjoyable.

Enjoy your new body, confidence and health

Printed in Great Britain
by Amazon